Your Skin, Your Care

Knowledge of skin cancer risk, recommendations for self-examination, and progress in medical therapy.

By

Shirley L. Brooks

Table of Content

Introduction

One kind of cancer that starts in the skin is called skin cancer. It happens when skin cells develop uncontrollably and abnormally. Although there are many different kinds of skin cancer, melanoma, squamous cell carcinoma, and basal cell carcinoma are the most prevalent types.

Prolonged exposure to ultraviolet (UV) light from the sun and tanning beds is the primary risk factor for skin cancer. Having fair skin, a history of sunburns, a family history of skin cancer, a compromised immune system, and exposure to specific chemicals are some other risk factors, though.

Typically, a skin inspection, biopsy, or other medical procedures are used to diagnose skin cancer. Depending on the kind and stage of the cancer, there are a variety of treatment options available, such as chemotherapy, radiation therapy, immunotherapy, and surgical removal.

An essential component of treating skin cancer is prevention. This includes avoiding tanning beds, using sunscreen, wearing protective clothes, and routinely checking your skin for any growths or strange changes to prevent excessive sun exposure. To improve skin cancer prognosis, early detection, and timely treatment are critical. See a medical expert if you observe any questionable changes to your skin.

The significance of prevention and awareness

To manage and lessen the effects of many health disorders, including diseases like cancer, awareness and prevention are essential. Their significance in skin cancer cannot be emphasized. The following justifies the need for preventive and awareness:

• Early Detection: If skin cancer is not identified in its early stages, it can be fatal, especially melanoma. initiatives to raise awareness encourage people to routinely check their skin and seek medical attention if they see any irregularities. These initiatives also teach people about the signs and symptoms of skin cancer. Better results and more successful treatment are achieved with early detection.

• Decreased Incidence: Excessive sun exposure and tanning bed use are frequently associated with skin cancer. Campaigns for public awareness educate individuals about the dangers of these behaviors, which can lower the incidence of skin cancer. Promoting sun-protection habits like donning hats, protective clothes, and sunscreen can also help reduce the risk.

• Preventing Complications: If skin cancer is not treated, it may result in scarring, deformity, and possibly the spread of the disease to other body parts. By practicing sun safety, one can help prevent these issues.

• Lower Healthcare Expenses: By raising awareness and implementing preventative measures, skin cancer can be avoided, which can result in significant healthcare cost savings. The cost of treating advanced skin cancer is higher than that of early identification and intervention.

• Better Quality of Life: People's quality of life can be enhanced by preventing and early detection of skin cancer. Preventing the need for major operations or intensive cancer treatments can help people keep their general health and looks.

• Public Health Impact: By lowering the overall illness burden, skin cancer prevention advances public health objectives. It can enhance a community's or society's general health and lessen the demand for healthcare resources.

• Education and Empowerment: By providing knowledge and information, awareness campaigns enable people. People are more likely to take proactive measures to avoid skin cancer when they are aware of the hazards and know how to protect themselves. Myths and misconceptions concerning tanning and sun exposure are also debunked via education.

• Encouraging Health-Related Behaviors: Awareness of skin cancer goes beyond simple skin care. It motivates people to take up healthy habits including eating a balanced diet, exercising, and abstaining from tobacco and excessive alcohol use. In general, these elements may be beneficial to health.

• Fostering Research and Development: Raising awareness frequently results in increased financing for studies on the prevention and treatment of skin cancer. Better preventative measures, therapies, and diagnostic instruments may result from this.

• Impact on Families and Communities: Prevention and awareness-raising can safeguard not only the individual but also the family and community. People may safeguard their loved ones and educate their communities by leading by example and sharing information.

In conclusion, raising public knowledge of skin cancer and promoting prevention is essential for preserving lives, lowering medical expenses, and enhancing general health. They enable people to take charge of their health and well-being, which promotes community safety and health.

Chapter 1: Recognizing the Skin

Since the skin is the largest organ in the body and involves many physiological processes, it is imperative to understand it. An outline of the skin's composition and operations is provided here.

The biggest organ in the body, the skin, acts as a barrier to protect internal organs from the outside world. It is composed of three primary layers, each with a different purpose:

• Epidermis: The epidermis is the skin's outermost layer and the primary defense against the outside world. It is comprised of multiple strata of distinct cells:

• Stratum Corneum: Dead skin cells, or keratinocytes, make up the outermost layer of the epidermis. New cells from the lower layers regularly replace these as they shed.

• Stratum Granulosum: A cell layer that produces keratin, a complex, fibrous substance that gives skin strength and waterproofing.

• Stratum Spinosum: These cells create keratin and contain spiny projections.

The bottom layer of the epidermis, known as the stratum basale (or stratum germinativum), is where new skin cells are formed. Melanocytes, which create the pigment melanin that gives skin its color, are also found in it.

• Dermis: Underneath the epidermis, the dermis is the middle layer of skin. It has a rich vascularization and a variety of structures and elements, such as:

• Blood Vessels: The dermis is home to blood vessels that provide the skin with nutrition and oxygen.

• Hair Follicles: The dermis contains hair shafts and sebaceous glands that secrete sebum or skin oil.

• Sweat Glands: Sweat glands are located in the dermis and control body temperature.

• Nerve Endings: The skin's sensory receptors in the dermis allow it to register pain, pressure, and temperature.

• Collagen and Elastin Fibers: These structural proteins strengthen and elasticize the skin.

• Subcutaneous Tissue (Hypodermis): Comprising connective tissue and fat cells (adipocytes), the subcutaneous tissue is the skin's innermost layer. It acts as padding and insulation, assisting in regulating body temperature and preventing damage to internal organs.

The thickness, texture, and properties of skin can fluctuate across individuals, and its structure varies depending on the area of the body. The development of skincare products, the diagnosis and treatment of skin disorders, and the avoidance of infections and skin-related illnesses like skin cancer all depend on understanding the skin's structure.

The importance of the skin in maintaining overall well-being

The skin is an intricate organ with several purposes and plays a significant part in general health. The skin serves the following primary purposes and is essential for preserving health:

1. Protection: The skin acts as a physical barrier to keep the body safe from harm from the outside. It is a barrier against chemicals, infections (such as bacteria and viruses), and physical damage. The epidermis, the outermost layer of skin, and the acidic properties of sweat and sebum (skin oils) aid in inhibiting the growth of pathogenic germs.

2. Thermoregulation: Body temperature control is dependent mainly on the skin. When the body is overheated, it can dilate blood vessels to release heat or constrict blood vessels to preserve heat in cold weather. Furthermore, sweating causes evaporative heat loss, which cools the body.

3. Sensation: We can engage with our surroundings by detecting different stimuli by sensory receptors in the skin. These receptors provide information about touch, pressure, temperature, pain, and other sensory experiences.

4. Excretion: The skin's sweat glands remove waste materials and maintain electrolyte balance. The body gets rid of extra heat and metabolic waste by sweating.

5. Immune Response: Immune cells found in the skin aid in the defense against infections and other illnesses. This immunological function is essential to stop diseases from entering the body through the skin.

6. Vitamin D Synthesis: The skin creates vitamin D when exposed to sunshine, an essential vitamin for healthy bones and calcium absorption. Sufficient levels of vitamin D are vital for general health.

7. Absorption: The skin can absorb materials like prescription drugs and topical therapies. Applications in medicine and cosmetics make use of this feature.

8. Sense of Identity: A person's physical appearance and sense of self are influenced by their skin tone, texture, and look. Keeping your skin healthy can improve your mental and self-esteem.

9. Hair and Nails: Although they are not a component of the skin, hair and nails are skin appendages. They offer additional defense and sensory capabilities and act as general health indicators.

The skin plays a variety of roles in overall health. Sustaining good skin is essential for general well-being as well as the appropriate operation of the organ. Because they can affect one's self-esteem and self-image, skin conditions or damage can substantially influence one's physical health, quality of life, and even psychological well-being.

Good skincare practices, shielding the skin from too much sun exposure, being hydrated, eating a balanced diet, and seeking medical attention for any irregularities or conditions relating to the skin are all key ways to preserve and improve the health of your skin. Additionally, improved general health and a higher quality of life can be achieved via knowledge of and attention to the skin.

Chapter 2: Definition of skin cancer

In the epidermis, the outermost layer of skin, skin cancer is the uncontrollably growing abnormal cells that result from unrepaired DNA damage that causes mutations. These mutations cause the skin cells to increase quickly and develop into cancerous tumors.

Although there are many different kinds of skin cancer, melanoma, squamous cell carcinoma, and basal cell carcinoma are the most prevalent types.

• Basal Cell Carcinoma (BCC): Basal cell carcinoma is the most prevalent kind of skin cancer. It usually manifests on skin regions, including the face, neck, and ears, that are frequently exposed to the sun. BCC often has a sluggish growth rate and a low propensity to metastasize. Open sores, red patches, pink growths, or shiny lumps are frequently its defining characteristics.

• Squamous Cell Carcinoma (SCC): Sun exposure is also the primary cause of Squamous cell carcinoma. It tends to grow more quickly than BCC and is the second most prevalent type of skin cancer. If SCC is not treated, it may spread to other body parts. It frequently manifests as elevated growths, open sores, or scaly red patches.

• Melanoma: The deadliest kind of skin cancer, melanoma is less common than BCC and SCC. It starts in the skin's melanocytes, which produce pigment, and if left untreated, it can quickly spread to other organs. Melanomas frequently arise from pre-existing moles or manifest as novel, atypical moles with atypical sizes, colors, and forms.

Reasons and danger signs

Exposure to ultraviolet (UV) radiation from the sun and artificial sources is the leading cause and risk factor for the development of skin cancer. The following are the main reasons and risk factors for skin cancer development:

1. Prolonged and cumulative exposure to ultraviolet (UV) radiation: The single most significant risk factor for skin cancer is UV radiation exposure. The DNA in skin cells is harmed by UV radiation from the sun and indoor tanning beds, which can cause mutations that can lead to cancer. Essential details about UV exposure are as follows:

The risk is increased by prolonged and intense sun exposure, particularly sunburns sustained throughout childhood and adolescence.

People working outside or spending much time outdoors are more vulnerable.

Using an indoor tanning bed exposes one to intense UV radiation, increasing skin cancer risk.

2. Fair Skin: Melanin, the pigment that offers some defense against UV ray damage, is less prevalent in those with fair or light skin. As a result, their chance of getting skin cancer is increased.

3. Family History: There may be a higher risk for those who have a family history of skin cancer, particularly melanoma. Genetic factors may influence skin cancer risk.

4. Personal History: Having a history of precancerous skin lesions, including actinic keratoses, or prior skin cancers can raise your chance of getting new skin cancers.

5. Sunburns: Sunburns are a risk factor for skin cancer, mainly if they occur frequently, especially in infancy or adolescence.

6. Specific Moles: Dysplastic nevi, or atypical moles, may more likely develop into melanoma. One risk factor is having a lot of moles, particularly odd moles.

7. Age: Growing older is associated with a higher risk of skin cancer, especially non-melanoma skin cancers (BCC and SCC). However, young adults are not exempt from the effects of melanoma.

8. Immune System Suppression: Skin cancer risk is higher in people with compromised immune systems, such as organ transplant patients or those with specific medical disorders.

9. Carcinogen Exposure: Skin cancer risk may increase as a result of occupational or environmental exposure to certain carcinogenic substances, such as arsenic.

10. Geographical Location: Residing in areas with high UV radiation levels, near the equator, or at more significant elevations can raise your risk of developing skin cancer.

11. Xeroderma Pigmentosum (XP): a rare hereditary condition that increases the risk of skin cancer by hindering the body's capacity to repair UV-damaged DNA.

It's crucial to remember that although these variables may raise the chance of developing skin cancer, they do not ensure it. To lower the risk and increase the likelihood of early detection and effective treatment, preventive measures such as sun protection (sunscreen, protective clothing, hats, and sunglasses), routine skin self-examinations, and early medical evaluation of any unusual skin changes or growths are essential.

Chapter 3: Signs of skin cancer

Depending on the type of skin cancer, there can be a wide range of unique manifestations as well as indications and symptoms. The following are some typical indicators and symptoms linked to various forms of skin cancer:

1. Open Sore: Basal Cell Carcinoma (BCC) BCC frequently manifests as a sore that oozes, crusts, or bleeds but does not heal. It might be glossy, transparent, pink, or red.

• Reddish Patch: A reddish patch that occasionally turns into a sore and may be irritating.

• Shiny lump: A tiny, pearly lump with a central depression and possibly visible blood vessels.

• Pink Growth: An elevated, pink growth with a crusty core and a somewhat rolled border.

• Scar-like Area: A pigment-free, white, yellow, or scar-like area.

2. Scaly, Crusted Patch of Squamous Cell Carcinoma (SCC): SCC frequently manifests as a painful or bleeding skin patch that is rough, scaly, or crusty.

• Open Sore or Ulcer: A sore or ulcer that either doesn't heal at all or heals only to reopen later.

• Thick, Red Nodule: A scaly, elevated red nodule with a firm texture.

• Wart-like Growth: This growth resembles a wart and may bleed or crust.

3. Melanoma: Melanoma is characterized by the "ABCDE" criteria for evaluating skin growths or moles and can present in various ways.

• Asymmetry: The size, shape, or color of one half of the mole or lesion differs from the other half.

• Border Irregularity: The mole's borders are notch- or scallop-shaped.

• Variation in Color: The mole comes in various colors, including brown, black, red, blue, and white.

• Diameter: Melanomas typically measure 6 mm, or 1/4 inch, in diameter, although they occasionally measure less.

• Changing: Over time, melanomas frequently alter in size, shape, color, or elevation.

Other indications of melanoma to be aware of include:

• New Mole or patch: The emergence of a novel, peculiar skin mole or patch.

• Itching or Pain: Melanomas may develop into painful, tender, or itchy lesions.

• Bleeding or Oozing: Melanomas have the potential to bleed or ooze.

• Spreading or structure Change: The mole or spot may take on an elevated appearance or take on a nodular structure.

It's crucial to remember that not every alteration or anomaly in the skin indicates skin cancer. However, seeing a medical practitioner for a full assessment is essential if you have any of the symptoms mentioned above or detect any strange changes in your skin. Success in therapy depends on early discovery, particularly in cases like melanoma, which, if left untreated, can be fatal. People who are at risk of developing skin cancer should perform regular self-examinations and have a dermatologist examine their skin once a year.

When to seek medical care

Seeing a doctor when you notice changes in your skin is essential to the early detection and prompt treatment of skin cancer. It is best to speak with a medical expert, ideally a dermatologist if you have any of the following symptoms or signs:

• New or Unusual Growth: You should have a new mole, spot, lump, or growth on your skin examined if it differs in appearance from your existing moles or if its size, color, or form is unusual.

• Modifications to Current Moles: A healthcare professional should inspect an existing mole if it begins to change in color, shape, size, texture, or elevation.

• Persistent Sores or Ulcers: You should get medical attention for any skin sore or ulcer that does not disappear in a few weeks. This is especially crucial for still oozing, bleeding, or crusting lesions.

• Bleeding or Oozing: It's a serious indication that has to be attended to by a doctor if a mole or skin lesion begins to bleed, ooze, or develop scabs.

• Itchiness or Pain: If a mole or lesion is constantly itchy or painful, you should check it out because skin cancer may be present.

• Quickly Growing Moles: A dermatologist should examine moles that multiply. Short-term changes may indicate a problem.

• Irregular Borders: Investigating moles or lesions with erratic, ill-defined, or scalloped borders is essential.

• Asymmetry: Moles that exhibit asymmetry—that is, where one half does not correspond with the other—should be checked out.

• Color Changes: A mole or lesion that shows variations in color or numerous colors may be a cause for concern.

• Family History: People who have a history of melanoma or other skin cancers in their family may be at a higher risk and ought to think about getting frequent dermatologist skin exams.

• Personal History: It's critical to schedule routine follow-up exams with your healthcare practitioner if you've previously had skin cancer.

• Painful Lesions: It is essential to examine any painful skin lesion, especially if it persists.

• Any Concern: Please don't hesitate to seek medical advice from a specialist if you have any concerns regarding a mole or skin lesion. Skin cancer diagnosis and identification must occur as soon as possible for optimal treatment and better results.

Recall that there are excellent treatment options for skin cancer, particularly for cases that are discovered early. Frequent self-scratches of your skin combined with yearly dermatologist skin inspections can aid in the early detection of possible problems. It is advisable to avoid caution and seek professional examination as soon as possible if you observe any of the signs mentioned above or symptoms.

Chapter 4: Diagnosis of Skin Cancer

Usually, a combination of techniques is used to identify skin cancer, such as a visual examination, dermoscopy, and, if required, a biopsy. A dermatologist, a medical professional with expertise in skin disorders, usually conducts the diagnostic procedure. This is a summary of the process used to diagnose skin cancer:

• Visual Examination: Examining the skin visually is the initial stage in diagnosing skin cancer. A dermatologist thoroughly examines the skin during this examination to look for abnormal growths, moles, or lesions. To detect possible indicators of skin cancer, such as uneven borders, color fluctuations, size changes, asymmetry, and other distinguishing characteristics, they employ their clinical experience. The patient's symptoms, such as discomfort, itching, or bleeding, may also be noted.

• Dermatoscope: A handheld device with a magnifying lens and a light source, the dermatoscopy is used in the dermoscopy procedure. Dermatologists can inspect skin lesions more closely with dermoscopy, making it easier to differentiate between benign and possibly malignant growths. It offers a closer look into the color patterns and structure of the lesion.

• Biopsy: A dermatologist will usually advise a skin biopsy if they believe a skin lesion could be malignant. A biopsy is the most reliable way to confirm a skin cancer diagnosis. There are various kinds of skin biopsies, such as:

• Punch Biopsy: A little, round piece of tissue is taken out from the suspicious location.

• Shave Biopsy: The top layer of skin is shaved off to get a sample.

• Excisional Biopsy: This method removes the entire lesion and some surrounding tissue.

• Incisional Biopsy: Only a part of the lesion is removed to facilitate evaluation.

• Pathological Examination: A pathologist, a medical specialist who analyzes tissue samples, assesses the biopsy sample after it is delivered to a pathology laboratory. The pathologist can ascertain whether cancer cells are present, classify the type of skin cancer (such as melanoma, squamous cell carcinoma, or basal cell carcinoma), and evaluate the stage and features of the malignancy.

• Staging and Additional Assessment: If a skin cancer diagnosis is confirmed, additional assessment may be required to ascertain the cancer's stage and extent. Imaging studies, such as CT, MRI, or sentinel lymph node biopsy, may be part of this to determine whether the cancer has progressed beyond the skin.

Treatment Planning: The dermatologist will create a customized treatment plan based on the staging and biopsy results, working with other medical professionals as appropriate. Surgical removal, radiation therapy, immunotherapy, chemotherapy, targeted therapy, or a mix of these methods are possible treatment options.

Skin cancer diagnosis and identification must happen as soon as possible to achieve the most significant results. It is advised to regularly examine your skin and see a dermatologist annually, particularly if you have risk factors for skin cancer. It's critical to get immediate medical assistance for a comprehensive evaluation and diagnosis if you detect any changes in your skin or have concerns about a specific mole or lesion.

The value of early identification

Like with many other forms of cancer, the significance of early identification in the case of skin cancer cannot be emphasized. There are essential, potentially life-saving consequences of early detection. The following list of factors emphasizes the significance of early skin cancer detection:

• Higher Cure Rates: Skin cancer is very treatable and frequently curable, mainly when discovered early. The likelihood of a complete recovery increases with early detection.

• Reduced Treatment Intensity: Treatment choices for skin cancer are typically less intrusive and aggressive when it is discovered in its early stages. Minimal invasive surgery or alternative interventions might be adequate to mitigate the patient's physical and psychological distress.

• Better Quality of Life: Early detection and treatment can prevent advanced skin cancer problems and disfigurement. It enables people to preserve their general quality of life, self-esteem, and beauty.

• Lower Treatment Costs: Compared to maintaining an advanced condition, treating skin cancer early on is typically less expensive. Both people and healthcare systems may benefit financially from this.

• Preventing Metastasis: If melanoma, a more dangerous type of skin cancer, is not detected in its early stages, it may spread to other organs. The prognosis can be improved by early identification, which can stop cancer from spreading to vital body components.

• Simplified Treatment Approaches: Shorter and less complicated treatment regimens are sometimes necessary for early-stage skin cancer. It reduces the need for prolonged therapy and several consultations.

• Lessened Emotional Stress: Receiving a cancer diagnosis can be pretty upsetting. Some of the psychological and emotional strain brought on by advanced disease and involved treatment plans can be reduced by early detection.

• Better Long-Term Survival: People who receive early detection are more likely to survive for a more extended period and have better general health, enabling them to lead fruitful and satisfying lives.

• Improved Public Health: Early detection programs and widespread knowledge can help identify skin cancer cases early, improving general public health and lowering the disease's burden.

• Educational and Preventive Opportunities: To further lower the prevalence of the disease, early detection programs frequently offer chances for public education regarding the significance of sun safety, self-examinations, and skin cancer prevention.

• Improved Prognosis: Early identification enables medical professionals to determine the exact type and stage of skin cancer, which helps them design the most suitable and efficient course of therapy.

People should regularly self-examine their skin, check for any unusual changes or growths, and seek expert review for any concerns to help with early detection. A dermatologist's annual skin examinations are also advised, especially for people who are more susceptible to skin cancer because of things like family history or prior skin cancer cases. Early detection, combined with sun protection and prevention, is the secret to effectively managing skin cancer and reducing its adverse effects on an individual's health and well-being.

Chapter 5: Available Treatments

Depending on the type of skin cancer, its stage, location, and personal circumstances, there are several treatment options. Melanoma, squamous cell carcinoma (SCC), and basal cell carcinoma (BCC) are the three primary forms of skin cancer. The following are typical courses of care for each:

1. BCC, or basal cell carcinoma:

Excision: Surgical excision is the primary treatment for bladder cancer. A margin of healthy tissue is removed along with the tumor. This is a very successful method for treating localized tumors.

Mohs Surgery: A specialist procedure called Mohs micrographic surgery is frequently utilized for BCC, particularly in regions where it is essential to preserve good tissue. Tiny tissue slices are removed and examined under a microscope to ensure that all cancer cells are removed.

Curettage and Electrodesiccation: In this technique, the tumor is removed with a curette, a tool shaped like a spoon, and any remaining cancer cells are destroyed by applying an electric current.

Cryotherapy: Liquid nitrogen is used to freeze the tumor during this treatment. Usually, it is applied to superficial BCCs.

Topical Medication: To treat superficial BCCs, the skin may be treated with specific creams or gels that contain drugs such as imiquimod or 5-fluorouracil (5-FU).

2. Cancer of the Squamous Cells (SCC):

Excision: SCC is frequently removed surgically. Together with the tumor, the surgeon eliminates a margin of healthy tissue.

Mohs Surgery: Mohs surgery might be suggested for SCCs at high risk or those situated in delicate cosmetic regions.

Curettage and Electrodesiccation: This technique applies to some SCCs, especially low-risk ones.

Radiation therapy: If surgery is not an option or if SCC has spread to neighboring lymph nodes, radiation therapy can be a possibility.

Topical Drugs: Topical drugs such as imiquimod or 5-fluorouracil (5-FU) may be utilized to treat certain superficial SCCs.

3. Malignancy:

Surgical Excision: The excision of the tumor and a margin of surrounding healthy tissue is the mainstay of treatment for melanoma. The melanoma's stage determines the depth and scope of the resection.

Sentinel Lymph Node Biopsy: To find out if cancer has migrated to neighboring lymph nodes, a sentinel lymph node biopsy may be necessary if the melanoma has a higher propensity for spreading.

Immunotherapy: To strengthen the body's defenses against melanoma, immunotherapy medications, such as checkpoint inhibitors (like pembrolizumab or nivolumab) and targeted therapies (like BRAF inhibitors like vemurafenib), are administered.

Chemotherapy: Due to the availability of more focused treatments, traditional chemotherapy is becoming less popular but is still helpful in the advanced stages of melanoma.

Radiation Therapy: In certain situations, such as when melanoma has metastasized to lymph nodes or is not surgically excisable, radiation therapy may be utilized.

Adjuvant Therapy: In high-risk instances, adjuvant therapy—such as immunotherapy or targeted therapy— may be suggested following surgery to lower the chance of recurrence.

Clinical studies: Patients with advanced or difficult-to-treat melanomas may be eligible to enroll in clinical studies.

It is noteworthy that the selection of a treatment plan is contingent upon the unique circumstances of each patient, encompassing the nature, extent, and site of the skin cancer. The development of treatment programs usually involves dermatologists, surgeons, oncologists, and other medical specialists working together. The effectiveness of treating skin cancer depends heavily on early detection and a timely diagnosis. It's crucial to go over treatment choices with a healthcare professional to find the best course of action for each patient.

Chapter 6: Risk mitigation and prevention

Reduced risk and prevention are critical in lowering the chance of skin cancer. The following are some crucial actions and behaviors that can reduce your risk and help prevent skin cancer:

1. Sun Shielding

Use Sunscreen: Even on overcast days, protect all exposed skin with a broad-spectrum sunscreen with an SPF (Sun Protection Factor) of at least 30. Apply sunscreen every two hours, or more often if you are perspiring or swimming.

Seek Shade: When the sun is at its highest, which is usually between 10 a.m. and 4 p.m., seek shade to protect yourself from the UV rays.

Put on Protective Apparel: Wear long sleeves, hats with wide brims, and UV-blocking eyewear to cover up your skin.

Steer Clear of Tanning Beds: Since sunlamps and tanning beds emit UV radiation, they raise the risk of skin cancer.

2. Frequent Self-Examinations of the Skin:

Self-examine your skin frequently to check for any changes in moles, birthmarks, or other skin growths. See a medical practitioner for an assessment if you observe anything unusual, such as newly developed or shifting moles.

3. Annual Visits with Dermatologists:

Make an appointment with a dermatologist for yearly skin examinations, mainly if you are more susceptible to skin cancer or have a family history of the disease.

4. Children's Protection:

Kids are more prone to the adverse impacts of the sun. Ensure they're adequately covered with clothing, sunscreen, and shade when outside.

5. Consider Your UV Exposure:

Rectangular surfaces that reflect light, like snow, sand, and water, can amplify UV rays. Up to 80% of UV radiation can be skipped by snow.

6. Utilizing sunscreen

All exposed skin, incredibly sometimes overlooked regions like the ears, neck, and feet tips, should be heavily covered in sunscreen.

7. Select a Sunscreen:

Choose a sunscreen that offers safeguard against both UVA and UVB rays. Seek out substitutes that are resistant to water when swimming or spending extended periods in the sun.

8. Prevent Serious Sunburn:

Seek shade, cover up, and use sunscreen to avoid being sunburned. A severe sunburn increases the chance of developing skin cancer, especially in children.

9. Safety Glasses:

Put on sunglasses that filter entirely UVA and UVB rays to shield your eyes from UV rays.

10. Drugs and Health Conditions:

Be advised that several drugs, illnesses, and medical procedures can make you more sensitive to the sun. If you have any concerns, speak with your healthcare professional.

11. First Time Detection:

The prognosis for skin cancer improves with early detection. Keep a close eye out for any changes in your skin, and get medical advice if you see anything unusual.

12. Limit Tanning: Steer clear of too much sun exposure and tanning, both artificial and natural. The term "healthy" tan does not exist.

13. Educational Programs: Take part in local initiatives to prevent and raise skin cancer awareness. Inform people,

including yourself, about the risks associated with UV rays and the value of preventive.

Adopting these risk reduction and prevention practices will help you drastically lower your risk of skin cancer. It's critical to remember that skin cancer is frequently avoidable and that early identification can enhance treatment outcomes. Make proactive measures to shield your skin from the sun's damaging rays, and motivate everyone around you to follow suit.

Chapter 7: Managing Cutaneous Cancer

Although having skin cancer can be a difficult and emotionally draining experience, a good quality of life can be maintained with the correct tools, support, and coping mechanisms. When dealing with skin cancer, bear the following essential points in mind:

1. Medical Attention and Therapy:

Observe your healthcare professional's prescribed course of action, schedule routine check-ups, and report any adverse effects or concerns.

2. Sun Shielding:

Keep shielding your skin from damaging UV rays. Use caps, sunscreen, and protective clothes, and adopt sun safety behaviors.

3. Emotional Assistance:

Seek out friends, relatives, or support groups for emotional assistance. It can be emotionally taxing to deal with a cancer diagnosis, but talking to others about how you're feeling might help them understand and offer comfort.

4. Self-Growth:

Make your general well-being and self-care a priority. Take part in relaxing and stress-relieving activities, such as yoga, meditation, or mindfulness.

5. Exercise and Diet:

Keep up a nutritious diet and, if you can, get frequent exercise. These routines can elevate your mood and help you feel better overall.

6. Self-Esteem and Body Image:

Your look may be impacted by skin cancer and its treatment. See a healthcare provider or counselor to improve your self-esteem and deal with any difficulties related to your body image.

7. Consistent Skin Exams:

Continue to self-examine your skin regularly, and notify your healthcare practitioner of any changes right away.

8. Become Informed:

Find out more about the treatment choices, possible side effects, and the particular type of skin cancer that you have. You can feel more in control and be able to make wise judgments if you know.

9. Establish Contact with Medical Experts:

Establish a helpful rapport with your oncologist, dermatologist, and other medical professionals. Clear and honest communication is essential to providing quality treatment.

10. Research Studies:

If suitable, consider participating in clinical trials to get access to innovative therapies and support cancer research.

11. Control Adverse Effects:

Take the initiative to control the side effects of treatment. Tell your medical provider about any pain or worries you may have.

12. Assistance Services:

Investigate supportive services that can improve your general well-being, such as social work, counseling, or nutrition counseling.

13. Education and Advocacy:

If you want to spread awareness and encourage others to participate in skin cancer advocacy and educational initiatives, consider participating.

14. Support for Family and Caregivers:

Include your caregivers and relatives in your trip. Their assistance is crucial and helps lessen the practical and emotional strains.

Managing skin cancer can be an enduring journey, so it's critical to approach each day with patience and awareness. Recall that you are not traveling alone on this adventure.

Many patients with skin cancer manage their condition well and go on to lead happy lives. Living with skin cancer can improve one's quality of life if one has self-care, a good outlook, and support from family, friends, and medical experts.

Chapter 8: Research on skin cancer and its prospects

Research on skin cancer is a dynamic area with continuous goals to enhance disease prevention, early identification, and therapy. The field of skin cancer research is expected to witness future developments in customized treatments, novel techniques, and technological breakthroughs. Here are some noteworthy study topics and anticipated products in the field:

Immunomodulation: Immunotherapy is being investigated for different forms of skin cancer and has demonstrated encouraging outcomes in treating advanced melanoma. Research is being conducted to find biomarkers that can predict treatment responses and to create more successful immunotherapies.

Targeted medicines: Research is currently being conducted on targeted drugs, which concentrate on particular genetic alterations and signaling pathways linked to skin cancer. Current research efforts are focused on finding novel targets and creating targeted treatments for skin malignancies other than melanoma.

Precision medicine: Personalized treatment plans that adjust medications based on a patient's unique genetic and molecular profile are becoming more popular. Treatment for skin cancer is anticipated to be significantly impacted by developments in precision medicine and genetic sequencing.

Early Detection Technologies: Scientists are developing cutting-edge tools to help identify skin cancer early. This includes enhanced diagnostic and imaging methods to identify skin cancer in its most curable and early stages.

Artificial Intelligence (AI): To help healthcare professionals identify patients more quickly and accurately, AI and machine learning are being used to evaluate medical images, such as dermoscopic images of skin lesions.

Sun Protection and Education: To raise public awareness of the significance of sun protection and early detection, research efforts are still concentrated on public health campaigns and educational initiatives. This includes programs designed to cut down on tanning bed use.

Research on prevention and sunscreens: Current studies look at encouraging sun-safe behavior, particularly in young adults and children, and how to make sunscreens more effective.

Cancer Vaccines: Research is still being done to create cancer vaccines, which include preventive shots for high-risk individuals and therapeutic shots for people who have a history of skin cancer.

Combination therapies: Research how to optimize treatment efficacy and reduce adverse effects by combining various treatment modalities, including immunotherapy, radiation, surgery, and targeted therapeutics.

Telemedicine: Patients can now obtain dermatological knowledge remotely with the growing use of telemedicine and teledermatology, which is particularly helpful in underserved areas.

Behavioral and Psychological Interventions: Studies on interventions aimed at promoting patients' psychological health and treatment compliance are being carried out.

Public Policy and Advocacy: By encouraging sun protection and increasing awareness, ongoing public policy and advocacy efforts aim to lower the prevalence of skin cancer.

It's crucial to remember that skin cancer research is advancing quickly and that new and improved methods for treatment, early detection, and prevention may be introduced in the future. In the fight against skin cancer, as with any medical research, cooperation between researchers, medical professionals, and advocacy organizations is crucial.

Conclusion

In summary, skin cancer is a severe health issue that has to be addressed and raised awareness of. To effectively tackle this condition, it is imperative to comprehend its risk factors, prevention tactics, early detection, and accessible therapies. Proactive measures, including sun protection, routine skin self-checks, and yearly dermatologist examinations, can lower a person's risk of getting skin cancer and increase the likelihood of an early diagnosis and successful outcome.

There are many different kinds of skin cancer, but the three most common ones are melanoma, squamous cell carcinoma (SCC), and basal cell carcinoma (BCC). Due to each variety's unique traits and growth and spread potential, early diagnosis and detection are crucial.

The cancer's kind, stage, and location will determine the best course of treatment, including immunotherapy, targeted medicines, and surgical excision. The chance of a good result increases with the early detection and treatment of skin cancer.

Skin cancer can be prevented and its risk reduced to the lowest possible degree by implementing preventative and risk-reduction measures. These measures include wearing sunscreen, having regular skin exams, and avoiding tanning beds. Promoting safe solar behaviors and early detection also requires education and awareness.

Although having skin cancer might be difficult, people can maintain a high standard of living with the correct medical attention, support networks, and self-care techniques. It's critical to continue managing the illness proactively on both a physical and emotional level.

Skin cancer research is still moving forward with encouraging advancements in immunotherapy, targeted medicines, precision medicine, and early detection technology. Future developments in skin cancer research could lead to better treatment, diagnosis, and prevention methods as knowledge and technology advance.

Finally, although skin cancer is a significant and common health issue, it is also a condition that can be successfully prevented, discovered, and treated, eventually enhancing the health and well-being of those who are at risk. This is made possible by education, awareness, and prompt action.